DARK MONEY:

The Hidden History of the Billionaires Behind the Rise of the Radical Right

By Jane Mayer |

Summary & Highlights with BONUS Critics Corner

Authored By

Summary Reads

FREE GIFT SPECIAL REPORT

The Tidiest and Messiest Places on Earth

When summarizing Spark Joy we made a special report about the Tidiest and Messiest Places on Earth! This report is a great supplement to that summary that is all about the virtues of being tidy.

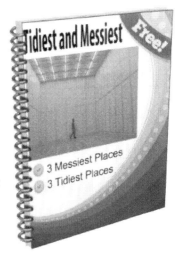

As our **free gift** for being a **SUMMARY READS enthusiast** we are happy to give you a special report about the **3 Most Messy** and the **3 Most Tidy** places on Earth.

Learn about everything from **Garbage Island** to Computer-Chip **Clean Rooms** (and, of course, everything in between).

Get your **free copy** at:

http://sixfigureteen.com/messy

ALSO: We will let you know about future Summary Reads titles so this is **win-win**! Enjoy your **FREE GIFT** and thank you for being part of the **SUMMARY READS** Family!

ISBN-10: 1523830174
ISBN-13: 978-1523830176

DISCLAIMERS

- Absolutely nothing in this volume is meant to constitute legal, financial, or medical advice nor are the opinions presented to be considered expert opinions.
- This volume is **NOT** meant to be a replacement for the original book, we believe our summation, key quotes and highlight analysis will increase interest in the complete book and not detract from it.
- In this volume, each particular detail is presented to the best of our knowledge and understanding of the recent book by Jane Mayer. If you think any of our analysis or summation is inaccurate **please email us** and we will correct it and publish an updated edition after we verify the inconsistency (levelproperty@gmail.com).
- Most importantly: absolutely no portion of this summation volume was written in a Starbucks.

CONTENTS

DARK MONEY – *SINGLE PAGE SUMMARY*

Dark Money is a deeply thought provoking book over the power of money on the American political system.

The first half describes many ultra-wealthy members of our society, how they came to this wealth, how they came to their political beliefs, and what kind of mark they want to make on society.

As the book goes on it enlightens the reader to the Supreme Court case *Citizens United* that opened the door for limitless financial contributions from any single corporation. This newfound freedom can lead ultra-wealthy billionaires to the mindset that they can work to create a desired result in any election.

This book will make you think about the political landscape of the United States and where your vote actually fits.

CHAPTER 1: RADICALS: A KOCH FAMILY HISTORY
(SUMMARY, HIGHLIGHTS & BEST QUOTES)

The fiercely libertarian billionaire Koch family owes part of its fortune to two of history's most infamous dictators: Joseph Stalin and Adolf Hitler.

Fred Koch was an oilman that invented an improved process for extracting gasoline from oil. This process would, eventually, land him in Russia and Germany building their crude oil refineries in the 1930s and the 1940s.

In 1930 Winkler-Koch began training Russian engineers and helping Stalin's regime set up fifteen modern oil refineries. This job paid Koch $500,000, which was a huge sum in the depressed economy of the United States and started him on his way to independent wealth.

After a two-year window of this job details go dark until about 1940 when Fred Koch founded a new company. The time that is missing is the time that Koch spent ample amounts of time flying to Germany to help Adolf Hitler and the Third Reich.

Under Fred Koch's leadership a refinery in Hamburg, Germany was finished in 1935 and it was one of the few German refineries that could produce high-octane gasoline needed to fuel fighter planes.

Koch continued his work in Germany and was supposed to be on ill fated the 1937 transatlantic flight of Hindenburg. A last minute change in plans delayed his arrival for the flight and caused him to miss the trip altogether.

During this time Koch had some pretty interesting political viewpoints. He suggests that, based on work ethic, that Germany, Italy, and Japan were the only stable countries in the world.

As World War II hit the United States Koch tried to enlist in the army. Instead his country asked him to make high-octane fuel for the American fighter planes, meanwhile, his Hamburg refinery became an important target in Allied bombing raids.

Working in the U.S.S.R. gave Koch concerns, eventually, about what communist would do to the United States. He joined the John Birch Society, an archconservative group best known for spreading far-fetched conspiracy theories about communism. In a speech in Kansas he asked a group of women afraid of becoming to controversial by joining the society whether or not they would be too controversial lying in a ditch with a bullet in their brain? All to show how bad the U.S. would be if communism were not taken seriously.

In 1964 Koch provided substantial support to Barry Goldwater and his right-wing bid for the presidential nomination.

Two of his four sons, Charles and David, became hard-line libertarians. Charles, in particular, voiced a deep-rooted hatred for America. He desired to see the current form of government uprooted.

Key Takeaways

The Koch family remembers Fred getting his first taste of how money can alter events when he routinely lost court cases, in his early business days, because the other side would pay a crooked clerk or a judge. "They believe justice can be bought and the rules are for chumps."

Fred Koch was a severe disciplinarian. Charles felt like he never could escape his father's rule until death. After his father's death Charles's goal was to achieve total control of the family's company.

YOU DECIDE: **@SummaryReads**

CHAPTER 2: THE HIDDEN HAND: RICHARD MELLON SCAIFE
(SUMMARY, HIGHLIGHTS & BEST QUOTES)

Richard Scaife, heir to the Mellon banking fortunes, was estimated at giving away over $1 billion in a fifty-year period on various philanthropy ventures. In 1999 the Washington Post claimed he was the "leading financial supporter of the movement that reshaped American politics in the last quarter century."

Politically Scaife shared a view with other influential conservatives that held the idea that the American civilization faced an existential threat from progressivism.

These men likened the fall of America to the fall of Carthage. Carthage's famous military leader, Hannibal, attacked Rome riding in on an elephant and was not backed up with support from the richer cities and people in North Africa, causing the fall of Carthage. This too, in their minds, would be the fate of the United States.

Through his father's work in the military and the Office of Strategic Services, forerunner to the CIA, Richard became increasingly aware of the threat of communism in America. This, along with the income tax, would be his priority in stopping for much of his life.

To make a difference Scaife supported presidential candidates. The Barry Goldwater loss to President Johnson was a huge blow, but Scaife rebounded by supporting Richard Nixon. Once Nixon's indictment from the Watergate Scandal hit the news Scaife began distancing himself from backing candidates.

In 1975 Scaife donated $195,000 to a new think tank called the Heritage Foundation. Over the next decade he gave over $10 million to this foundation and by the late 90s he had given over $23 million. This foundation prided itself on instilling deep conservative views in the American mainstream; their ideals and methods won Scaife over causing him to be, by far, their largest contributor.

Key Takeaways

The founder of the Mellon family fortune was Judge Thomas Mellon. In the late 1880s he began to worry that this enormous wealth would lead to his heirs not working. When someone doesn't have to work and are "freed from the necessity of exertion they begin to degenerate sooner or later in body and mind."

In order to escape mass taxation from war preparation in World War II and the hated income tax many of the ultra-wealthy put their wealth in a private foundation. These foundations are required to give 5% of their wealth to public charities, but also receive tax breaks from that giving. This enables the wealthy to maintain their fortunes and get breaks on the income taxes they are already paying. In 2013 over $800 billion American dollars was protected in private foundations.

YOU DECIDE: @SummaryReads:

CHAPTER 3: BEACHHEADS: JOHN M. OLIN AND THE BRADLEY BROTHERS
(SUMMARY, HIGHLIGHTS & BEST QUOTES)

John Olin was a proud graduate of Cornell. In 1969 a bloody incident of black protesters took place on campus. The protesters demanded an independent black studies program and the investigation of a cross burning outside a dormitory that had several black female residents.

This "liberal" agreement agreed to by the university's president prompted Olin, who had several buildings named after his family at Cornell, to take his philanthropy in a bold, new direction.

With his corporation facing numerous court battles over contamination in several states John Olin directed his lawyer to enlist his fortune in the battle to defend corporate America. At first the foundation funneled money into the same think tanks that Scaife supported. Soon his focus turned to academia.

Under the leadership of the newly appointed of William Simon, childhood friend of Olin, The Olin Foundation started funneling money into lesser known colleges where conservative money was welcome. Quickly Simon and the foundation noted this as a losing strategy and learned they needed to infiltrate the prestigious schools, especially the Ivy League.

What emerged from that idea was the "beachhead" theory. The aim was to establish conservative cells, known as beachheads, at the most influential schools in the country. The key was to stay away from department heads, rather, find likeminded professors whose own power and influence could grow if financed correctly.

Key Takeaways

By the time the John M. Olin Foundation spent itself out of existence in 2005, it spent half of its total assets of $370 million bankrolling the promotion of free-market ideology and other conservative ideas on the country's campuses.

YOU DECIDE: **@SummaryReads:**

CHAPTER 4: THE KOCH METHOD: FREE-MARKET MAYHEM
(SUMMARY, HIGHLIGHTS & BEST QUOTES)

As The Koch refineries faced many decades of legal battles over contamination in the workplace, Charles Koch kept his focus on his mission: to unceasingly advance the cause of liberty.

The Koch family fought against government regulations. In order to protect their "liberties" they would lie and falsify gas emissions.

They paid fines to several different regulatory boards across many different states for dumping hazardous chemicals and other byproducts into protected environmental areas.

This reckless unwillingness to follow governmental protocol came to a boiling point in 1996 when two Texas teenagers burned to death after starting a truck that caught fire from a gas leak of a nearby eroded Koch pipeline.

The wrongful death case had the father of one of the teenagers requesting $100 million in damages. With Koch's history of cavalier safety practices in the court's eyes the jury demanded Koch Industries pay $296 million in damages, at the time the largest wrongful death award on record.

Key Takeaways

The United States government found a deep secret in Koch Industries that they had stolen $31 million in oil from native tribes in Kansas. Koch explained that producing oil was an inexact science and very difficult to measure accurately. A study showed that no other company struggled with measurement quite like Koch Industry.

YOU DECIDE: **@SummaryReads:**

CHAPTER 5: THE KOCHTOPUS: FREE-MARKET MACHINE
(SUMMARY, HIGHLIGHTS & BEST QUOTES)

A part-time professor pursing a doctorate at NYU and teaching an Austrian economics course at Rutgers hit Charles Koch up to fund the study of Austrian Economics. Charles pledged $150,000 into the study.

By the late 1980s that part-time professor, Richard Fink, had become Charles Koch's main political lieutenant.

Previously the Kochs had disdained conventional politics, but under Fink's guidance became powerful Republican donors.

Fink led Koch to approach his giving in the political landscape into three categories: campaign, lobbying, and philanthropic. This approach allowed the Koch family to use its vast wealth to influence policy and politics from a variety of different directions.

Key Takeaways

After suffering humiliating losses in the courts and Congress, the Kochs began to retool their approach not to just to business but politics as well.

YOU DECIDE: @SummaryReads:

CHAPTER 6: BOOTS ON THE GROUND
(SUMMARY, HIGHLIGHTS & BEST QUOTES)

In 1984 Koch founded Citizens for a Sound Economy. In its first years Koch was easily the largest donor giving almost $8 million in the first 7 years.

As CSE (Citizens for a Sound Economy) grew it became a breeding ground for major corporations to get some political pull.

In 1993 CSE successfully attacked President Bill Clinton's proposed tax on fossil fuel. Later on it became accused of being a rent-a-cause since companies like Exxon and Microsoft would donate large sums of money and soon after CSE would espouse lobby many beliefs that would directly help its largest contributors.

In 2003 CSE split. The reason why is still foggy even to those closest to the split. No matter the exact reason it was about control and Charles Koch wanted CSE to fight for the causes that directly benefited Koch Industries.

Key Takeaways

The creation of Citizens for a Sound Economy was Phase 2 of Richard Fink's plan to benefit Koch Industries.

YOU DECIDE: @SummaryReads:

CHAPTER 7: TEA TIME
(SUMMARY, HIGHLIGHTS & BEST QUOTES)

Many believe that the Tea Party was started by spontaneously by Rick Santelli's rant on CNBC when he denounced Obama's plans to bail out homeowners and then proclaimed that he was going to have a tea party in July, in Chicago.

In 1991 the CSE promoted a massive re-enactment of the Boston Tea Party in North Carolina to protest tax increases. This, and other planned protests, has led Charles Koch to face many questions about his involvement in the Tea Party.

What faced President Obama was a new form of political power. No longer was it a campaign to drag mud on opposing candidates, rather, people with enormous wealth that could get a rise out of the public without having to show their face.

The Tea Party movement is less grass roots and more "Astroturf" with the amount of ultra-wealthy backers supporting it. To many the Tea Party was less spontaneous and more set up through decades long movements that led to this far right concept.

Key Takeaways

Though the reports of the spontaneity were not entirely wrong but to say that was the beginning in its entirety is far from the truth. Since FDR almost all Democratic presidents have faced attacks from the far right.

YOU DECIDE: @SummaryReads

CHAPTER 8: THE FOSSILS
(SUMMARY, HIGHLIGHTS & BEST QUOTES)

Climate change seemed, in 2008, as a bipartisan issue. Both presidential candidates, Obama and McCain, voiced publicly the need to reduce the pollution caused by burning fossil fuels.

Once President Obama took office he didn't realize the great impact that money would have in fighting climate change. He used a bipartisan strategy called cap and trade. This model for reducing emissions forced the oil and gas companies to pay for the pollution.

This idea had worked greatly with industries that caused acid rain and it felt like an easy way to reduce fossil fuel pollution. What supporters of cap and trade did not take into account was the enormous wealth that would be behind stopping these pollution practices.

The problem for the oil, gas, and coal industry was the by 2008 climate change presented such a dastardly future that if the world were to stay within the carbon emissions that would make the atmospheric temperatures tolerable, 80% of fossil fuel in reserve would have to stay unused.

Koch and his organizations tore into global warming and worked to debunk every single report that would cause a need in reduction of emissions.

Key Takeaways

Koch and others in his circle would be negatively financially impacted by such a bill, so Koch brought together a Who's Who in the oil, gas, and coal industry to financial back the fight against cap and trade.

YOU DECIDE: **@SummaryReads:**

CHAPTER 9: MONEY IS SPEECH: THE LONG ROAD TO CITIZENS UNITED
(SUMMARY, HIGHLIGHTS & BEST QUOTES)

On January 21, 2010 the Supreme Court made a landmark decision. For over a century corporations were limited in how much money they could give to help a candidate get elected. In a 5-4 decision the Supreme Court overturned that limit as long as the money wasn't just given to the candidate, rather, split between third party groups that either supported or opposed a candidate.

The co-founder of Amway, Richard DeVos Sr. was one ultra-wealthy industrial leader that was tired of the restraints of the old laws that limited financial contributions to $5,000 a year.

Amway has spent millions in fighting the IRS and the Federal Trade Commission over tax rights, Social Security, and the idea of calling Amway a pyramid scheme. This caused a deeply rooted desire to protect big business just like Charles Koch.

The DeVos family, before the 2010 Supreme Court case, sent millions every year to pro-Republican think tanks and organizations. Saul Anuzis once remarked that there is no Republican president or candidate in the last 50 years that did not no the DeVoses.

The DeVos family is credited with being a major reason this Supreme Court decision came down.

Key Takeaways

The Supreme Court's ruling that took off the financial cap placed on corporations giving to candidates (Citizens United) was given based on the attorney's ability to get the justices to accept that corporations have the same rights to free speech as citizens.

YOU DECIDE: **@SummaryReads:**

CHAPTER 10: THE SHELLACKING: DARK MONEY'S MIDTERM DEBUT, 2010
(SUMMARY, HIGHLIGHTS & BEST QUOTES)

With the Citizens United decision opening up new frontiers for the ultra-wealthy dark money was going to make an impact.

The election of Scott Brown in Massachusetts was a coup for the Republicans. Massachusetts had not elected a Republican to the Senate in 38 years. To make matters worse for the Democrats this was the seat held by the recently deceased Ted Kennedy.

Because the Supreme Court lifted restrictions in giving to different third party funds Brown was able to outspend his opponent by over $3 million.

The House vote that brought the Affordable Care Act into realization caused the dark money billionaires to rethink their attack. They knew one thing had to be done; the House of Representatives must go back to the Republicans in the mid-term elections.

Koch and other ultra-wealthy businessmen use social welfare groups to fund their money for campaigns. These groups, under law, do not have to disclose the identity of private donors. Through these groups Charles Koch was able to raise $75 million for the mid-term elections.

Sean Noble, head of a wealthy social welfare group broke down the Democratic seats he felt the GOP could win in the election. Then, through an excel spreadsheet, he ordered these seats in order of most likely to go Republican. Based on that spreadsheet he and Koch began to divide the money between the Republican candidates.

Key Takeaways

The Scott Brown vote turned the tide in the Senate not allowing the Democrats to stop a Republican filibuster because it lowered them below the 60 votes needed to stop such an act.

YOU DECIDE: **@SummaryReads:**

CHAPTER 11: THE SPOILS: PLUNDERING CONGRESS
(SUMMARY, HIGHLIGHTS & BEST QUOTES)

The Republican coup of the mid-term elections brought the Koch brothers into the heart of GOP power. For years the Koch family was considered "libertarian losers" and now with the new dark money funds they were at the heart of D.C.

The new Congress say many, now indebted, Representatives that had loyalty to the Koch family. Many of these Congressmen would champion the causes espoused by the Koch family for deregulation and big business climate change protection.

YOU DECIDE: **@SummaryReads:**

CHAPTER 12: MOTHER OF ALL WARS: 2012 SETBACK
(SUMMARY, HIGHLIGHTS & BEST QUOTES)

With the Citizens United decision in their back pocket the Koch brothers set out to win what Charles called "the mother of all wars," the 2012 Presidential Election.

The first potential candidate that the Koch's set their eye on was Paul Ryan. He declined. The dark money backers were afraid that Mitt Romney would not appeal to the common masses and though he was a serious candidate decided to look elsewhere.

After working to get Chris Christie run Christie reluctantly decided that 2012 was not his year. Mike Pence was the next man on Koch's radar and he chose not to run also.

Romney, wanting Koch support, changed his views on two major issues: climate change and the budget. In a speech, where David Koch was present, Romney laid out a plan very similar to Paul Ryan's.

Romney faced irreparable damage by the other Republican candidates, for instance, Newt Gingrich. The plan these other candidates used to defeat Romney in several states was the blueprint for President Obama to attack as well. The Koch's always wanted a common face to there billions. Romney would prove far to out of touch to reach the common masses.

Key Takeaways

Mitt Romney's inability to relate to the common man was one of the reasons that most dark money backers are never seen. These ultra-wealthy billionaires prefer to allow more common men to be the upfront speaker and let their money dictate where the common man goes.

YOU DECIDE: **@SummaryReads:**

CHAPTER 13: THE STATE: GAINING GROUND
(SUMMARY, HIGHLIGHTS & BEST QUOTES)

Though the 2012 presidential election did not go the way of the Koch family, they would still categorize it as a success. The REDMAP plan created by Ed Gillespie was tried out in North Carolina. Through congressional district redrawing Republicans were able to win more seats in the State Congress than the Democrats despite receiving fewer popular votes.

Key Takeaways

The REDMAP plan was a plan that dark money backers felt could inspire real change in the political field. But winning each state it would garner enough Republican control to do the work that these backers felt needed to happen.

YOU DECIDE: **@SummaryReads:**

CHAPTER 14: SELLING THE NEW KOCH: A BETTER BATTLE PLAN
(SUMMARY, HIGHLIGHTS & BEST QUOTES)

Conservatives, dark money backers especially, had an image problem. Polls began to show that only 38% of the public felt that Republicans cared about them. As the GOP sought to restore order from the Obama reelection they had to start with image.

The Koch's took one major step "If the 1 percent wanted to win control of America, they needed to rebrand themselves as champions of the other 99 percent."

One Koch Industry employee remembered that after the 2012 election if you stated you worked for Koch you may as well stated you worked for the devil, that is how low Charles Koch's image had fallen.

Koch and other billionaire families believed that the problem wasn't the content of the message but the packaging. The free-market viewpoint of Koch and the conservatives appeared to be pro-1% and anti-middle class. The GOP had to work to show that this was simply not the case.

These messages were misconceptions that could be clarified rather than rendered useless and thrown away. In an interview with the USA Today Charles Koch rebuffed the idea that he espoused these ideas of tax reform, deregulation of major pollutant laws, and other conservative platforms were not to pad his bottom dollar, but for the good of all man.

Key Takeaways

The public had decided that the Democrats were the "helping-the-poor guys" while the Republicans were the money guys. If conservatives wanted to win they had to change that image on both ends.

Charles Koch used to tell a joke when he was a child that never got a laugh out of anyone - when asked for how he would split a treat with others he would say "I just want my fair share - which is all of it."

YOU DECIDE: **@SummaryReads:**

Bonus Feature: Critics Corner

The main problem with her book may lie, not so much in its execution, but in the premise of its slant. Money is by no means a phenomenon of the conservative right.

George Soros funnels millions of dollars through several hundred political organizations. He recently pushed for the death of the U.S. dollar in favor of the globalist Banker controlled Special Drawing Rights (SDR).

Jeffrey Epstein is a wealthy New York financier, Democratic fundraiser and political donor. He recently made headlines for using underage prostitutes to curry influence with the Clintons and Prince Andrew.

Anti-Koch brother rhetoric may very well be justified, but it certainly is not unique to this book. They've had many documentaries and televised hit pieces made against them, even inspiring a diatribe on Aaron Sorkin's Newsroom.

While massive donations and political investment may garner detrimental results, danger is subjective. Where you stand on the political spectrum may determine which politically active financial entities pose the greatest threat.

The most sinister of these groups are most likely the faceless and the nameless industrial complexes that regularly fund and influence both political parties.

For example, pharmaceutical companies, defense contractors and the banking cartel exercise a monstrous sea of influence on both sides of the political landscape, with both Democrats and Republicans.

While this bitter truth may not fit into a convenient left-right paradigm, its prevalence is as far-reaching and its implications are insidious. Ms. Mayer may have gained more legitimacy if she at least addressed this greater epidemic.

While we have tried to give Ms. Mayer the benefit of the doubt and chosen our criticism carefully, some reviewers are not so reserved in their feedback. The worst review we could find was:

> "One main problem with this book is that a salacious journalist with absolutely NO understanding of economics is writing on a subject far out of her depth."

That might be a little harsh, but it does ring true when reading through her vitriolic tome.

However, there have been many critics that have received her work warmly (usually from left leaning journals). The Times Book Review sums up the sentiment of those that loved her work in its review of the book:

> "The book is written in straightforward and largely unemotional prose, but it reads as if conceived in quiet anger. Mayer believes that the Koch brothers and a small number of allied plutocrats have essentially hijacked American democracy." - *Times Book Review*

FURTHER READING

Are you ready to quickly absorb the main points and highlights of the next best seller? Check out the other great summaries from *Summary Reads*:

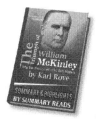 Karl Rove's latest book, *The Triumph of William McKinley: Why the Election of 1896 Still Matters* is a great read, but it is a LONG book. We have already read it and summarized it for you so pick up a copy and enjoy:

http://amzn.com/B018Y0POJY

Brian Kilmeade's latest best-seller, *Thomas Jefferson and the Tripoli Pirates,* is a fascinating story about a forgotten war. Get the summary today:

http://amzn.com/B018B8FFWK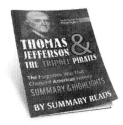

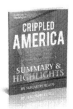 Crippled America is Trump's latest book and we have the top summary on the market:

http://amzn.com/B017QT0IMM

The over 900 page best-seller *Destiny and Power* is a great book but not everyone has the time for the whole book. Check out our summary and save hours: http://amzn.com/B019D70GI6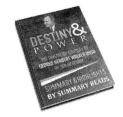

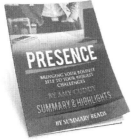
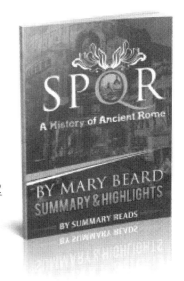

FREE GIFT SPECIAL REPORT

The 10 Strange Deaths of Vladimir Putin

While there is plenty of shady dealings going on in the United States, don't think foreign countries are any different. For example, in Russia what seems to keep happening to opponents of Vladimir Putin?

As our **free gift** for being a **SUMMARY READS enthusiast** we are happy to give you a special report about some of the mysterious and <u>strange deaths</u> that have befallen Mr. Putin's enemies.

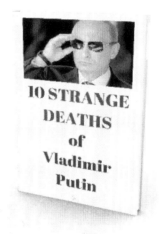

Plane crashes, multiple stab wounds and **radioactive sushi** are just a few of the misfortunes that have befallen those who opposed the Russian President.

Get your free copy at:

http://sixfigureteen.com/summaryreads

<u>ALSO</u>: We will let you know about future Summary Reads titles so this is **win-win**! Enjoy your FREE GIFT and thank you for being part of the SUMMARY READS Family!

EXTRA FREE GIFT SPECIAL REPORT

The Tidiest and Messiest Places on Earth

When summarizing Spark Joy we made a special report about the Tidiest and Messiest Places on Earth! This report is a great supplement to that summary that is all about the virtues of being tidy.

As our **free gift** for being a **SUMMARY READS enthusiast** we are happy to give you a special report about the **3 Most Messy** and the **3 Most Tidy** places on Earth.

Learn about everything from **Garbage Island** to Computer-Chip **Clean Rooms** (and, of course, everything in between).

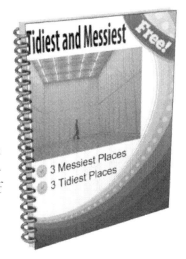

Get your **free copy** at:

http://sixfigureteen.com/messy

ALSO: We will let you know about future Summary Reads titles so this is **win-win**! Enjoy your **FREE GIFT** and thank you for being part of the **SUMMARY READS** Family!

33566369R00022

Made in the USA
San Bernardino, CA
05 May 2016